HATHA YOGA, A

This is a simple course of Hatha Yoga containing basic exercises for busy people. It has been specially compiled for safe use by Westerners and is a valuable guide for the training of the physical body as an instrument for the true man, the spiritual Self. The author also includes simple exercises for meditation and mind control and advice on personal hygiene and diet, all of which form part of the ancient science of yoga, aiming at the development and expression of man as an integrated being.

Wallace Slater is a scientist who has spent more than forty years in the study and practice of yoga as part of his daily routine of life.

HATHA YOGA
A SIMPLIFIED COURSE

by

WALLACE SLATER

THE THEOSOPHICAL PUBLISHING HOUSE LTD

68 GREAT RUSSELL STREET, LONDON WC1B 3BU

ADYAR, MADRAS INDIA   WHEATON, ILL. U.S.A.

© Theosophical Publishing House (London) Ltd.

First edition 1966
2nd and revised edition 1977

ISBN 0 7229 5062 4

Illustrations by courtesy of
Quest Books, a department of
The Theosophical Society in America.

Printed in Great Britain by
Fletcher & Son Ltd., Norwich

SUMMARY OF THE LESSONS

Page

Introduction
      Hatha Yoga and other forms of yoga   1

Lesson 1

A   Hygiene   6
B 1 Relaxation posture (shavāsana)   7
C 1 Basic breath   7
D   Thinking selectively   8

Lesson 2

B
(i ii iii) Preparatory stretching   9
C 2 Head cleansing breath (kapāla bhāti)   10
C 3 Bellows breath (bhastrikā)   11
C 4 Throat cleansing breath (ujjāyi)   12

Lesson 3

A   Further hygiene   14
C 5 Empty breath (rechaka)   16
C 6 Full breath (pūraka)   16

Lesson 4

A   Diet   18
B 2 Back-stretching posture (paschimottan-āsana)   20
D   Meditation   22

Lesson 5

A	Controlled thinking affects bodily re-actions	24
B 3	Twist posture (ardha-matsyendrāsana)	25
D	Meditation	28

Lesson 6

A	The nervous system	29
B 4	Plough posture (halāsana)	30
B 5	Bow posture (dhanurāsana)	32
D	Regular daily meditation	33

Lesson 7

A	The chakras	35
B 6	Cobra posture (bhujangāsana)	35
B 7	Hand and foot posture (padahastrāsana)	37
C 7	Prana breathing	39

Lesson 8

B 8	Simple cross-legged posture (sukhāsana)	41
B 9	Advanced cross-legged posture (siddhāsana)	43
B 10	Lotus posture (padmāsana)	44
C 8	Chakra breathing	45

Lesson 9

B 11	Shoulder stand (sarvāngāsana)	49
B 12	Abdominal uplift (uddīyānā bandha)	52
C 9	Cooling breath (sitakari)	52
C 10	Another cooling breath (sitali)	53
D	General notes on meditation	53

Lesson 10

	How to use the system	57
B 13	Pelvic posture (supta-vajrāsana)	57
B 14	Locust posture (shalabhāsana)	59
B 15	Head stand (shīrshāsana)	61
B 16	Peacock posture (mayūrāsana)	63
D	Meditation to solve a problem	63
	Typical daily programme	64

In each lesson the instructions are grouped thus:

A. General
B. Postures
C. Breathing
D. Meditation

PREFACE

There have been many books published on yoga and more recently a fair number has appeared on Hatha Yoga. This *Simplified Course* was prompted by requests for an ordered course of training in the form of lessons which could be spread over a period of 20 to 40 weeks. It was also required that the exercises should be critically selected to include only those which could be readily used by people in the western world without risk and without the need for personal instruction. Lastly, the course was required by busy people who could only spare a short time each day for its practice.

The selection of material has been based on a wide study of yoga literature, personal tuition from several teachers and over forty years' practice of yoga in general, including those aspects of Hatha Yoga which have been found of value in looking after the well-being of the physical body as an instrument for man's true inner spiritual Self. It is hoped that the reader will regard this course as supplementary to a serious study of yoga in general and of Raja Yoga in particular.

V. W. SLATER

INTRODUCTION

THE RELATION OF HATHA YOGA TO OTHER FORMS OF YOGA

Yoga is a process by which the laws of Nature are intelligently and deliberately applied to daily life in order to realize in full self-consciousness, one's identity with the Supreme. It is based on the theory that the real man is not his body. The real self is a spirit which uses the body as an instrument. The literal translation of the Sanskrit word, yoga, is "union", and it is taken to mean union of spirit and matter. Since spirit is regarded as belonging directly to Universal Consciousness, it is associated with the higher principles of man and his eternal self. The body on the other hand is impermanent, non-eternal. Thus the union implies a dominance over matter (the body and its lower associations) by spirit.

The seven principal schools of yoga are:

Hatha which is based on control of the physical body to open it to the cosmic energy by breathing and physical exercises.

Laya which works on the psychic centres to awaken the primordial cosmic energy of the individual (Kundalini).

Mantra which makes use of the repetition of certain words and phrases to steady the mind.

The above three work by operating from the outer periphery of consciousness to an inner centre.

The following three proceed as from the inner Self outwards:

Jnana which seeks to effect union of higher and lower by a change of thought, resulting from the attainment of deep understanding of the working of the laws of the universe (Yoga of Knowledge).

Bhakti which seeks to effect union by a change of one's emotional consciousness through devotion to an ideal (Yoga of Devotion).

Karma which seeks to effect union by control of one's actions from the inner spiritual Self (Yoga of Action).

All the above six are embraced in:

Raja Yoga, the earliest and most scientific treatment of the subject of self-transformation for the attainment of union with the Real, the Eternal

This course on Hatha Yoga is based on the principle that all forms of yoga begin with Hatha and finish with Raja, a statement which requires qualification. Raja Yoga seeks to control changes in consciousness, and by this control to rule the lower vehicles. Hatha Yoga seeks to control the vibrations of matter, and by this control to evoke the desired changes in consciousness. This latter imposes a great strain on the comparatively intractable material of the physical body, sometimes leading to damage of the very organs whose activity has been stimulated.

The Hatha yogi in theory proceeds in consciousness from the physical to mental to spiritual, but in practice often aims at psychic experience. The Raja yogi is advised to work from the spiritual through the mental to the physical, ignoring the psychic.

The reason why a limited form of **Hatha Yoga**, however elementary, should accompany any of the other forms of yoga is because the physical body cannot be neglected or ignored. It is wise to live simply and to ensure a balanced living at all levels. The unwise practice in the past in India, and by some westerners, was in those Hatha Yoga practices which reverse the process of evolution by regaining conscious control by the will of those bodily functions, such as the action of the heart, control of body temperature, digestion, etc., which should no longer concern the waking consciousness and which have been relegated to the "sub-conscious", the automatic nervous system.

The exercises given in the course have been selected from the very wide range of Hatha Yoga practices to avoid such over-emphasis on the physical organs. In following this course it is recommended that the exercises be used only as supplementary to a more spiritually-based form of yoga. Thus it is wise to establish a spirit of meditation whatever the form may take. Some people cannot meditate in a formal manner, but everyone can make of life a meditation in the sense of identifying his thinking with a spiritual object. This gives power to create from the spirit through the mind into physical forms. Since the physical body is an important vehicle during incarnation, some consideration must be given to its care and preparation as an instrument for the spirit.

Control of the physical body is therefore not an end in itself but a means to an end. Each should work this idea out for himself with the idea that our sub-conscious is the past, our conscious the present, while our super-conscious is a state to be attained in the future. Meditation on the ideal one wishes life to assume will help that attainment, and this should be kept in mind while going through this course.

This course is on Hatha Yoga, but since this Introduction has mentioned other yogas, the student should note that Hatha, Laya and Mantra Yogas alone will not result in self-realization: Hatha can be a useful supplement when carefully directed; Laya can result in too early an awakening of uncontrolled psychic centres; Mantra can also be a useful supplement but here also care is required.

To sum up: Hatha Yoga is that form which deals with the care, health and well-being of the physical body. This should be regarded, not as an end in itself, but as the preparation of a well-balanced nervous mechanism with which to work. Let this preparation be accompanied by development of the highest principles so that the true inner spiritual self may be able to manifest through our thoughts, feelings and actions in the outer world.

The instructions and exercises in this course are grouped under four headings:

A. General
B. Postures
C. Breathing
D. Meditation

This classification is used in each lesson for easy reference and because all four procedures should be followed at the same time. Textbooks usually give all the postures in one or more chapters and then all the breathing exercises in another chapter, but for a planned course of training it is necessary to proceed along the four lines in each lesson.

A. *General.* This section will deal with general advice such as personal hygiene and diet, an important aspect of Hatha Yoga.

B. *Postures.* These are physical exercises which are not muscular development exercises such as are used for the training of athletes and they cannot be called "physical jerks". They are postures for bending and stretching the trunk and limbs. The Indian term is āsana which literally means a seat.

C. *Breathing.* This is an important aspect of all yoga. The Indian term is prānāyāma which is taken to mean the voluntary control of breathing, from prāna, the breath, or more generally the life-principle.

D. *Meditation.* This covers all aspects of mind control from concentration of thought (dhārana or exclusive attention to one idea), through meditation (dhyāna or continued attention taken beyond the plane of sensuous perception) to contemplation (samādhi, the final fulfilment or state of ecstasy, complete self-possession).

We are now ready to begin yoga training. Follow the instructions slowly and carefully, making sure that you can carry out the exercises comfortably and without strain, before passing to the next lesson.

LESSON 1

A. General

Hygiene

In addition to the normal daily hygiene the nasal passages should be washed out once a day, never more than twice. Warm water is cupped in the hand and sniffed up each nostril and then expelled by blowing out, first of one nostril and then of the other. Doing this twice should be sufficient to clear the nasal passages first thing every morning. Avoid violent blowing of the nose as this may affect the duct leading to the ear.

Some people may find that water alone may cause pain in the mucous membrane, but with continued practice this will gradually disappear. However, if preferred, one can use a solution of normal saline which works without any irritation. To make normal saline dissolve one level teaspoonful of salt in one pint of water. This has the same salt content as tears.

This regular cleaning of the nasal passages is an excellent preventative for colds, sore throats and nasal catarrh.

It is important to ensure that all elimination processes are working efficiently and this must include the skin and the lungs. A friction bath using a wet towel over the whole body will help the skin to eliminate poisons, and efficient breathing is necessary for the lungs. The tongue should be cleaned with the toothbrush as well as the teeth.

For sleeping, warm bedclothes are necessary, but these should be of light weight.

The amount of drink taken at meal-times should be reduced. It is better to drink between meals, or before or after the meal.

B. Postures

(1) *Relaxation posture* (shavāsana)

Lie flat on the back with the feet slightly apart and relax muscle by muscle from the head downwards, terminating the exercise by contracting or stretching each muscle group also from head to toe.

Begin the exercise by breathing in and out slowly and deeply a few times. Then let the whole body go limp. Feel each muscle group relax: eyebrows, mouth, neck, shoulders—and so on to the toes.

Then follow the same course but now tensing each muscle group.

Finally have a good overall stretch.

C. Breathing

(1) *Basic breath*

Lie flat on the back with hands on the diaphragm, i.e. just below the ribs. *Breathe in* through the nose slowly and as deeply as possible. As the lungs fill slightly press on the diaphragm to force air into the chest. Fill with air the lower, middle and upper parts of the lungs in that order. Then *breathe out* as slowly as you breathed in, through the nose. Gently draw in the abdomen at the end of the breathing-out.

Do this six times, finally expelling the air quickly.

D. Meditation

Think selectively. Choose what you are going to think about, then think seriously about it. This is not just an early morning exercise, this is for the whole day. Try to make all thinking, during the day, more definite and clear.

In particular think optimistically.

LESSON 2

A. General

After being in a stuffy or smoky atmosphere, cleanse the lungs with the "head cleansing breath" as given below in section C (exercise 2).

B. Postures

The best time for relaxation and other posture exercises is early morning before breakfast. If this is not possible then do them in the evening before the evening meal.

Prepare for the yoga postures, to be given in later lessons, by preliminary stretching. In lesson 1 it was pointed out that these postures (āsanas) are bending and stretching exercises, and the need to go carefully without strain was also emphasized. This is most important and therefore the only exercises recommended in the early lessons, other than the relaxation posture, are general ones as follows:

i. Sit on the ground with the legs straight and slowly bend the trunk with the hands stretching towards the feet. The movement must be a slow stretch without any jerks, and do not worry if, at this stage, you cannot bend very far.

ii. Lie flat on your back and stretch out the legs and arms, right out as far as possible.

iii. Just lie relaxed on back or side and stretch and yawn as if just waking up.

In each of the above stretching exercises finish by a momentary extra stretch, hold and then let go.

C. Breathing

Begin the following three breathing exercises with care. If they cause giddiness it is because you are trying to make too rapid progress. Begin by doing each exercise once only, then twice and gradually work up to six times at the daily session.

Have a short rest after each exercise, taking a few normal breaths before the next exercise.

(2) *Head cleansing breath* (kapāla bhāti)

Sit cross-legged on a rug or cushion on the floor or "Egyptian fashion" on a chair. The cross-legged position is natural in countries like India and some westerners prefer it. There are several ways of crossing the legs, but at this stage just take whatever method comes really easy, with the spine as nearly vertical as possible. This will be referred to as the "Lotus pose". The "Egyptian pose" is on a chair with legs and feet together and spine upright. It is better not to lean on the back of the chair, but to let the hands give whatever support is necessary by resting them in the lap.

For this exercise, in either position, rest the hands on the knees with the palms up.

Breathe in and out (through the nose) several times slowly. Then take one long slow breath, followed by a quick expulsion (through the nose). Do this slow in and quick out six times. The air should be expelled in say one second, noting that the expulsion should be forced from the muscles of the abdomen.

It may be necessary to hold a handkerchief in front of the nostrils during the early practice. If the nasal passages have been cleared by the method given for the daily hygiene in lesson 1, section A, there should however be no trouble here.

(3) *Bellows breath* (bhastrikā)

Lotus or Egyptian pose with the left hand across the lap, palm up.

Use the right hand to control the nostrils, the thumb on the right nostril and the third finger on the left nostril.

Prepare by *exhaling through the right* nostril, using slight pressure of the finger to close the left nostril. Then *inhale through the right* nostril. Then *exhale through the left* nostril followed by *inhaling through the left*, then *exhaling through the right*.

The timing should be reasonably quick but full. Take twice as long to exhale as to inhale.

The complete cycle should be repeated three times, making six breaths, thus:

> out right,
> in right, out left,
> in left, out right,
> in right, out left,
> in left, out right,
> in right, out left,
> in left, out right.

(4) *Throat cleansing breath* (ujjāyi)

Pose as for head cleansing breath, C 2.

According to the Sanskrit literature on Laya Yoga, this breath is to fill the body with prana from throat to heart (*Serpent Power*, Arthur Avalon).

Exhale completely.

Inhale through the nostrils, but with the windpipe slightly constricted. One way of learning to do this is to breathe in so as to make a snoring noise. Another is to pronounce the sound "ing" and hold that back-of-the-mouth position while breathing in. Still another way is to breathe in through the nose with the mouth open; to make sure that the air comes through the nose the back of the mouth has to be closed and this produces the desired result. Breathing-in like this produces a restricted intake such as one sees with a child or a dog when it cannot have its own way.

Then exhale slowly with the windpipe fully open, taking twice as long as for the inhaling. The exhaling may be through the nostrils, but some people prefer to exhale through the mouth.

Do this cycle six times.

Exhaling through the mouth has the advantage of thoroughly clearing the throat passage, so that the complete breath clears the passages between the nose and throat.

Sanskrit Terms

Throughout this course the Sanskrit terms for the exercises have been given, in brackets. There is no need to use these, but they will help for reference purposes when consulting books on yoga, some of which use only Sanskrit terms.

Prana. This Sanskrit term literally means "breath" but has the wider meaning of "cosmic life manifesting at all levels". Thus it is the life principle which vitalizes our thinking, feeling and acting. At the physical level it energizes the whole nervous system. Breathing takes in oxygen to feed the whole circulatory system with that element necessary for the release of energy. In yoga it is understood that prana is similarly absorbed by the vital counterpart of the dense physical body. This vital "background" is sometimes called the etheric body. For further details see *The Etheric Body* by A. E. Powell.

LESSON 3

This course has been planned on the basis of two weeks for each lesson. Students will determine their own rate of progress, but it is more important to proceed slowly rather than to try to rush it.

A. General

Further Hygiene

The following are additional notes on personal hygiene.

Teeth: toothpicks are recommended to be used, to supplement the toothbrush, to clear debris from crevices between the teeth.

Tongue: brush as far back as possible.

Ears: syringe about once a year with water no hotter than 105°–110° F.

This is the temperature of a very hot bath. Use a rubber ball syringe (or plastic rubber substitute).

Nose: rinsing with lukewarm water each morning, as recommended in lesson 1, can cure catarrh far better than medicinal sprays.

Eyes: when travelling (bus or train) relax the eyes for several minutes by focusing on the horizon. Then change by focusing on something quite close, and then back to the horizon. During the day the eyes can be relieved of strain by palming them for 2 to 3 minutes, i.e. resting the eyes on the palms of the hands with the elbows on the table. *Do not press* on the eyeballs. Splashing closed eyes with cold water is very refreshing, psychologically soothing and physically invigorating.

B. Postures

We are not yet ready for more definite exercises. Just keep on with the relaxation posture and the preliminary exercises of lessons 1 and 2. The breathing must be right before going on to the specific postures (āsanas) which will begin in lesson 4.

C. Breathing

Additional to (1) *Basic breath* (See Lesson 1)

It is now necessary to introduce some control over the rate of breathing during the exercises. Most people breathe too fast and too shallow. Sitting in a chair note your normal rate by counting seconds. You will probably find that you take 2 to 3 seconds to breathe in, and 2 to 3 seconds to breathe out. This means 12 to 15 respirations per minute; some medical books give 15 to 18 per minute.

When the mind is quiet, as in meditation, the breathing tends to become slower and deeper. It is therefore recommended that during the breathing exercise period the rate should be gradually reduced. For a few days extend the time for in-breathing to 4 seconds, and the same for out-breathing. Then go to 5, then 6, and finally 7 seconds, giving a final respiration rate of only 4 to 5 per minute instead of the normal average of 15.

It is very important to take several days or weeks to reach the final slow rate, and then it should only be done during the exercise period or during meditation. Even then it should not be kept up if it causes any feeling of strain.

This slow rate can also be used for the other breathing exercises except where a quick rate is specified.

(5) *Empty breath* (rechaka, *meaning "out breathing"*)

Lotus or Egyptian posture with hands folded on the lap.

Take a few deep steady breaths. Then exhale fully, i.e. breathe out counting 7; then continue to breathe out to the limit, finishing with a "puff-out" through the lips. The lungs will now be as empty as possible, so follow by normal breathing again.

Do not repeat this more than once during the exercise period. Many people find it quite sufficient to do it just once only, without a repeat.

We have called this the "empty breath". Some books refer to it as the "lung cleansing breath", and recommend the whole breathing-out to be by a series of short puffs until the lungs are empty. Either method may be used.

(6) *Full breath* (pūraka, *meaning "filling-up"*)

This is the reverse of empty breath.

Lie flat on the back.

Breathe steadily three or four times.

Then breathe out fairly strongly followed by breathing *in* by small vigorous sniffs until the lungs are full.

Do not repeat more than once.

During all the breathing exercises it helps to think that you are taking in life-vitality (prana), during the in-breathing.

You now have a routine series of breathing exercises which should be used daily and in the order given:

(1) Basic
(2) Head cleansing
(3) Bellows
(4) Throat cleansing
(5) Empty (or lung cleansing)
(6) Full

These exercises will take 8 to 10 minutes and will have a vitalizing effect on the whole system, at the same time bringing a sense of calm and quiet to the mind. Medically they can relieve chronic bronchitis and other nose, throat and lung complaints—well worth the 10 minutes a day.

D. Meditation

Read the short note under D in lesson 1 again, in preparation for the next lesson.

LESSON 4

A. General

Under this heading we have thus far dealt with personal hygiene. It is now time to review *eating habits*. The following advice must be adapted to the individual. For example, the statement that it is better to drink 1 to 2 hours before a meal may not suit everyone. Hatha Yoga teachers in India are, however, very strict and dogmatic in their dietary rules. We consider that it is better to adapt these rules to the individual's type of body and his circumstances.

i. Cut down drinking at meal-times. Drink an hour or so before or after a meal.

ii. *How* to eat is more important than *what* to eat. Chew all food thoroughly and eat less. Starch and sugars are digested in the mouth. If time for the midday meal is short, make this a light meal and have the heavier meal when there is time to eat leisurely.

iii. Do not eat immediately before or after exercise or immediately after physical work or a hurried walk.

iv. Do not eat when there is emotional tension. In such a case take time to calm down.

v. A large hurried breakfast is bad. If in a hurry, eat less rather than more quickly.

vi. Do not eat just because it is meal-time—unless you feel you need food.

vii. With regard to *what* to eat, a vegetarian diet is recommended, that is, no meat, fish or poultry. Natural foods are preferred to processed food, but some people cannot digest salads after midday. Honey, milk, vegetables and fresh fruit make a good basis, but there must be adequate protein such as eggs, cheese, legumes or nuts taken in moderation. It is the excess protein taken by meat eaters that puts the extra load on their kidneys and liver.

viii. For drinks, fruit juices are best, but *freshly made* tea, even if strong, will cause no harm. The same applies to coffee in moderation, although many people cannot take this because of its over-stimulating effect.

ix. Although milk is a drink, it can be sipped with the meal, because it is really a food. Do not drink milk as a drink, i.e. pouring it down, but "eat it" slowly.

x. Music is helpful at meals. It tends to encourage leisurely eating, especially if eating alone. This is better than reading a study book. If you must read at mealtimes, choose light reading.

B. Postures

We are now ready for specific posture exercises. The stretching you have been doing has prepared the way, and the exercises given in lesson 2, page 9, can be discontinued.

Remember that each posture (āsana), except the relaxation one, is a prolonged stretch or contraction. Never jerk into position, but put on the stretch slowly, and maintain it as long as possible without strain. This may mean doing it for only 10 seconds or for as long as 5 minutes. Stop as soon as you feel that an extra second would be a strain.

(2) *Back-stretching posture* (paschimottanāsana)

This first stretching exercise is a basic one to stretch the spine, shoulders and arms.

i. Lie flat on your back, legs together, hands resting on the thighs. Slowly raise the head and trunk until you are sitting with the back upright and the hands still resting on the thighs with the elbows bent. Then slowly lower the back and head to the ground again. Do this only once or twice for the first few days and then proceed as follows.

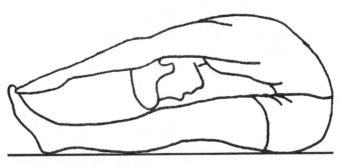

PASCHIMOTTANĀSANA

ii. Lie flat on your back as above but, as you slowly raise the head and trunk, stretch the arms forward instead of letting the hands rest on the thighs. Then *exhale* slowly while bending forward until your hands touch your toes, but keeping the legs straight. If you cannot touch the toes when you begin you will be surprised how easily you can do so after a few weeks. On no account must you strain yourself; just go as far as you can, a little more each day. After the forward bend, slowly reverse the movement to lie flat on your back again, while *inhaling*.

iii. When the above (ii) has been achieved, modify it by beginning with the arms above and behind the head, so that, as you raise the trunk to an upright position, you also raise the arms vertical above the head. Then continue to bend forward with trunk and arms until the hands touch the toes.

iv. At a still later stage bend forward and touch your knees with your face, at the same time touching your toes with your hands. This is the full posture. Hold this fully bent posture for say 10 seconds and then gradually reverse the movement—first to spine-upright and then to flat-on-your-back, *inhaling* as you do so and relax.

Later you may be able to hold the bent-forward stretch for up to 1 minute, but do not exceed this. The **final full posture need only be done once daily, at the exercise time.**

From this first stretching posture you will realize why this system of Hatha Yoga postures is one for stretching rather than "jerking". All movements are carried out slowly, and the full stretch maintained for a few seconds, and then the whole body is relaxed.

C. Breathing

Continue with the breathing routine established so far, and tabulated in lesson 3; these six breathing exercises should be done before the back-stretching posture.

D. Meditation

Hatha Yoga, in its limited form, does not include meditation. It is a system for cultivating a controlled physical body by stretching postures, breathing exercises and attention to diet and hygiene, as given under the headings B, C and A in this course. Its wise application, however, includes the practice of meditation as found in the other yogas, particularly Raja Yoga.

The following quotation from *Great Systems of Yoga* by Ernest Wood gives a good picture of the attitude of Hatha yogis to meditation:

"Samādhi, the highest practice of yoga, is conceived in a very material manner in the Hatha Yoga books. The idea is that the yogi in samādhi is uninfluenced by anything external, because the senses have become inactive, and he does not even know himself or others. Although the *Gheranda Sanhitā* says that the samādhi involves union of the individual with the supreme Self (Parātman) so that 'I am Brahma and no other; Brahma am I, without any sorrows; I am of the nature of fundamental existence, knowledge and bliss, always free and self-supporting,' it also prescribes, for the attainment of this, various mudrās or physical practices, such as that of turning the tongue into the nasal cavity and stopping the breath, the theory being that all you need to do is to cut off contact with this world, and the other state will be there."

This course will therefore not deal with the practice of meditation in detail as it is assumed that this "Simplified Course of Hatha Yoga" is supplementary to the practice of Jnana, Bhakti, Karma or Raja Yoga as mentioned in the Introduction. The student is therefore referred to such books as the following for more detailed advice on meditation:

Meditation for Beginners, J. I. Wedgwood.
Meditation, A practical course, Adelaide Gardner.
Concentration, Ernest Wood.
Concentration and Meditation, Christmas Humphreys.

The notes given here are for general use to encourage the student to follow up this course by meditation and other yoga practices which can lead to true self-realization. On the other hand it is realized that many people, well trained in meditation and the "more spiritual" yogas, may only be using this course as supplementary, on the principle that a healthy body is the best instrument for self-expression.

At this stage therefore, the following suggestions will help to link up Hatha Yoga exercises with the practice of meditation.

Have a positive attitude to everything you do or think about. Negative attitudes invite failure.

Control your attitude by always looking at the optimistic side. Be constructive in your thinking.

Have a plan for each day, but do not be a slave to the plan.

Feel friendly to everyone—forgive their weaknesses.

Remember that worry, anxiety and fear will not solve any of your problems.

Learn to withdraw into an inner privacy of mind even in the thickest crowd.

When concentrating your thought on a problem, give particular attention to relaxing the muscles round the forehead, eyes and mouth.

LESSON 5

A. General

Controlled thinking affects bodily reactions.

It is now recognized that thoughts and emotions have an effect on the hormone balance of the body. Hormones are chemical substances produced mainly by the endocrine glands and released into the blood stream. These hormones influence and control the functioning of the various organs of the body and are normally produced and released in just the right amounts to suit the bodily requirements with regard to age, type of activity, climate, etc. Certain emotional or mental activity can alter the rate of secretion to help the person through a period of mento-emotional stress, but the amount, whether reduced or increased, may be bad for his general welfare. Certain organs may be stimulated to activity beyond their natural capacity, with consequent collapse. Also the glands themselves may lose their fine control.

These results have been recognized by teachers of yoga throughout the ages without necessarily knowing the biochemical reason. Hence their emphasis on control of mind and emotions, and on the principle of non-attachment.

The following are some of the rules for control of man's occult centres (chakras) and, through them, of his glandular system:

i. Be temperate in all things. Avoid extremes.

ii. Take a more detached view of life, neither over-elated by success nor depressed by failure. Avoid excitement in either direction.

iii. Think about other people rather than about yourself. Do not be a cause of injury to others. Be compassionate.

iv. Have a goal which you can hope to attain. If it is too high it will result in discouragement if you fail. Frustration is a self-imposed injury. If you succeed you can then raise the standard, step by step.

v. Think before you act. A wrong thought can be rectified more quickly than a wrong action.

The above comments might have been given under section D, Meditation, but they have been given in the general section because they are directed towards the improvement of "personal hygiene", stretching this term to include the glandular system.

B. Postures

(3) *Twist Posture* (ardha-matsyendrāsana)

The literal translation of the Sanskrit word is half (ardha) Matsyendra (this being the name of the Indian Rishi who developed this āsana), and so some books call it the "half-twist".

i. Sit on a rug on the floor with the legs stretched out in front, trunk erect. Bend the left knee to bring the left heel near the top of the inside of the right thigh. The sole of the left foot is now against the inside of the right thigh. The left knee will be pointing outwards to the left.

Now, bring the right leg over to the left and place the sole of the right foot on the floor just to the left of the left thigh. The right knee will then be near the left armpit.

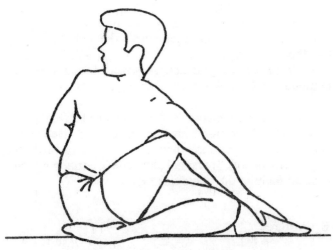

ARDHA-MATSYENDRĀSANA

ii. Place the right arm across the small of the back, palm outwards. Bring the left arm to the right of the right thigh, left hand on the right calf or grasping the right ankle. (If this is not possible, then just hold the right knee with the left hand.) Stage i has locked the pelvis in an anti-clockwise position. Stage ii has twisted the torso and shoulders clockwise. Hold this twist (pelvis anti-clockwise, shoulders clockwise) for a few seconds, trying to maintain the maximum twisting position without any jerking.

Then return to the original position, legs straight out in front and repeat the twist in the opposite direction.

Do this twist posture once only in each direction and hold each twist for a few seconds only, never more than 30 seconds. Later the neck should also be turned as far as possible in the same direction as the shoulders, thus achieving a twist of the whole spinal column, first in one direction and then in the other.

It is most important for this posture not to use too much strain, especially at the beginning. As with all the postures you must feel your way gradually. Just see how far you can go without discomfort, and you will find you can go farther each week.

You now have two postures to be done after the six breathing exercises. It is quite sufficient to do each posture only once at a time, the twist being once in each direction. If done properly this is ample. The relaxation posture, which is the only non-stretching one, should be done before the breathing exercises.

C. Breathing

Keep up the six breathing exercises as tabulated in lesson 3, and not forgetting to breathe deeply and slowly.

D. Meditation

The place of meditation in Yoga is outlined in my small book *Raja Yoga, A Simplified and Practical Course.*

The different yogas do not depend for essentials on one another, and each can be worked separately. There is, however, some benefit by taking them in sequence. Provided one does not stop at the level of the physical body, it can be useful to begin with the body for "to despise the body is to despise life". Having purified the body by attention to diet and hygiene, and having attuned it to express its cosmic significance and rhythm by the postures and breathing exercises, the mind must be brought into the practice.

First restraint of mind, i.e., drawing away the mind from all interests of the senses. Then the contemplation of the "Deity" ensouling the yogi's higher Self. And finally the union of the individual with the Universal Life.

Thus control of the mind is the whole ideal of all yoga.

Let these thoughts inspire you to include meditation in your daily practice so that the mind, the heart (devotion) and the body may be united with the Eternal, the flame of which the individual Self is a spark.

If you are not familiar with the practice you will probably find *Meditation for Beginners,* by J. I. Wedgwood, the most convenient book to use while going through this Hatha Yoga Course.

LESSON 6

A. General

The Nervous System

Yoga acts particularly on the nervous system. This is of great benefit in western civilization where there is so much strain. The practice of meditation calms the jumpy restless mind. In Hatha Yoga the postures (āsanas) strengthen the nerves. Breathing exercises harmonize the whole system and feed the nerves with oxygen.

Osteopathy is a form of medical treatment specially developed to help the nervous system, the spine being the main channel for the bundles of nerve fibres, which convey impulses between the brain and the rest of the body. These impulses may be sensory or motor. A reflex action is an automatic motor response from a sensory impulse which does not need to go to the brain, but can be generated from a complex in the spinal cord itself. It is therefore important that the vertebrae of the spine should be kept in good alignment. This does not mean "in a straight vertical line". The spine must be allowed its natural curves, e.g. neck forward, not army-fashion vertical, nor should the chest be projected forward military fashion. The natural curves may be seen on any good diagram of the side view of the human skeleton. The Hatha Yoga postures may be regarded as a form of self-osteopathy.

29

B. Postures

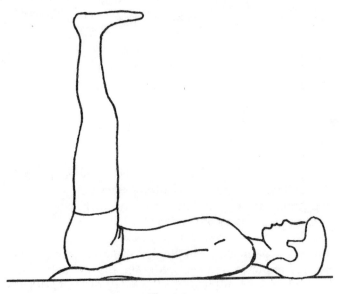

HALĀSANA (i)

(4) *Plough Posture* (halāsana)

i. Lie flat on your back, hands at the sides. Raise the legs very slowly, knees straight, until they are 90° from the floor, i.e. the legs vertical with the soles of the feet parallel to the floor. This should take about 10 seconds. Then hold this for 2 to 3 seconds.

ii. The body is then slowly raised to swing the legs over the head until the toes touch the floor behind the head. The knees must be kept straight and the palms of the hands flat on the floor. At this stage the back will not be quite vertical.

You will not complete this posture at the first or second attempt, but go as far as you can.

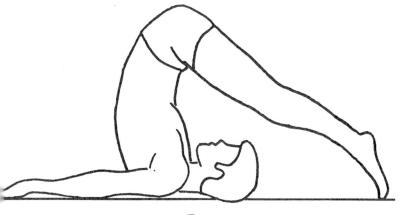

HALĀSANA (iii)

iii. When you can fairly comfortably complete stage ii, with the toes just touching the ground, slide the toes forward from the head to bring the spine really vertical and try to bring the thighs, legs and feet as near to one straight line as possible. In the complete exercise, stage iii follows immediately after stage ii. The aim then is to hold stage iii for up to 30 seconds, but only once at the daily practice.

Then slowly reverse the process and relax flat on the floor.

Obviously this posture must be progressed very slowly to avoid undue strain on the back. Do not worry if you cannot go beyond half-way between i and ii for some time. It is surprising how easy it becomes after a few months, and it is well worth the effort.

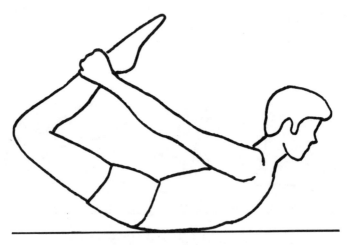

DHANURĀSANA

(5) *Bow Posture* (dhanurāsana)
This is the reverse of the plough.

Lie face downwards. Bend the legs at the knees and grasp the ankles with the hands (Right hand for right ankle, left hand for left ankle). Pull the feet well down towards the back.

When the above can be done easily, slightly open the

space between the knees and pull hard on the ankles to lift the thighs off the ground and, at the same time, to raise the head and shoulders, looking straight ahead. Hold this for 5 to 15 seconds only and do once only during the daily exercises.

For the period of this lesson

(*a*) do the six breathing exercises as tabulated in lesson 3, followed by

(*b*) the four postures: back-stretching,
twist,
plough,
    and bow.

D. Meditation

It was pointed out in lesson 4 with further comments in lesson 5, that Hatha Yoga, in its limited form, does not include meditation as a mental exercise, but rather as an exercise to suppress the senses. The preliminary practices suggested in lessons 1 and 4, and in the general section of lesson 5, will have helped to give you a relaxed mind so that you should be facing daily life with a feeling of calm equanimity. Those suggestions were of a general nature and were to be practised throughout the day as a background to Hatha Yoga.

In lesson 4 it was stated that this course will not deal with meditation in detail, and the would-be yogi was referred to specialist books on the subject. At this stage in Hatha Yoga training we strongly recommend the introduction of a regular daily meditation of a more definite character than the general practices mentioned above. You may already be doing this, and some will have had many years' experience long before taking this Course. In any case the meditation should follow the breathing and posture exercises.

If, however, you have no experience of meditation you could now begin by having a short period of mental relaxation after the Hatha Yoga exercises. Just sit cross-legged or "Egyptian fashion" (as described for the breathing exercise 2 in lesson 2), close the eyes, breathe naturally and calmly. Feel at peace with yourself and with the world. Say to yourself, "My body is not the Self. I withdraw my consciousness from my body". Pause and feel the meaning of the above.

Then say to yourself, "I am not my emotions". Pause and feel the emotions as calm sympathy for others.

Then say "I am thinking these thoughts, but the Self is higher than the mind. I will control my thoughts". Pause and feel that relaxed sensation when thought itself ceases.

Then take a few deep breaths and feel the life of the higher Self flowing into the mind, the emotions, the body—and rise with the sense of being in control of your vehicles of outer consciousness.

The whole exercise should not take longer than 10 minutes at this stage. Even 5 minutes can be quite useful.

LESSON 7

A. General

The Chakras

At this stage most Indian schools would introduce a study of the occult centres of the body, the *chakras*. There are seven such centres: the crown on the top of the head (sahasrara), the brow between the eyebrows (ajna), the throat at the front (vishuddha), the heart (anahata), the solar plexus (manipura), the spleen (svadhishthana) and the root at the base of the spine (muladhara).

For further details you are recommended to read *The Chakras* by C. W. Leadbeater, *The Etheric Double* by A. E. Powell, and *Introduction to the Chakras* by P. Rendel. For advanced study see *Serpent Power* by Arthur Avalon.

B. Postures

(6) *Cobra posture* (bhujangāsana)

Lie face down on a rug or folded blanket, chin on the ground, hands palms down at shoulder level, elbows sticking up. Keep the legs together on the ground and stretch them well back, stiff and straight with the soles of the feet up, but feet still on the ground.

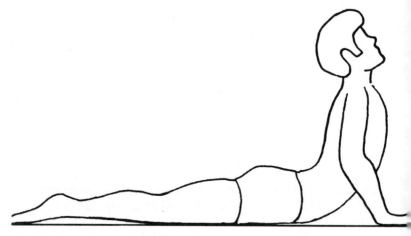

BHUJANGĀSANA

Now raise the head slowly as high as possible, chin jutting forward to the fullest extent. Then try to lift the chest off the ground, assisted by pressing down with the hands on the floor. Try, however, to do as much as possible with the back muscles. Keep the body from toes to navel on the ground, curving up from there.

It is called the cobra posture (bhujang means cobra) because the position is in imitation of a cobra about to strike.

Hold the final position for a few seconds, increasing the time with practice up to one minute. Then slowly and smoothly return to the original face-down position.

Most important—do not strain the back muscles by a jerking and wrenching action.

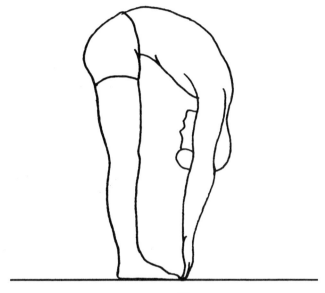

PADAHASTRĀSANA

(7) *Hand and foot posture* (padahastrāsana)

Stand erect with the legs together. Breathe in raising the hands above the head, arms straight. Then, while *exhaling* fully, bend the body forward and downward, to bring the hands towards the toes. Try to touch the toes with the fingers, keeping the knees straight.

The ultimate aim is to touch the knees with the nose, and to place the hands flat on the ground, but it will probably be some time before you can do this. In any case it depends on the individual's bone structure, i.e. the length of the leg bones relative to the spine and arms.

Hold the posture for 5 seconds, later increasing to 30 seconds. Then raise the body to the upright position while inhaling and bringing the arms above the head. Exhale as you lower the arms to the sides.

You will note the similarity of this posture to the back-stretching posture (No. 2 of lesson 4). If you are pressed for time you can omit one of them. One is a vertical exercise while the other is horizontal so that each has a distinct use, but the hand and foot posture is the more effective.

You have now been given seven postures and should begin to see the plan for your daily routine. They have been introduced in the course in an order suited to the final programme. This is arranged so that one posture naturally leads to the next one, as follows:

	back stretching	(No. 2)
	twist	(No. 3)
and	*plough*	(No. 4) on the floor.
Then	*bow*	(No. 5)
and	*cobra*	(No. 6) on the floor face down.
Followed by	*hand and foot*	(No. 7) standing up.

The above are the six basic postures which should be done daily, in that order, after the six breathing exercises. The relaxation posture (No. 1), not being a stretching one, should precede the breathing exercises. A form of meditation should then follow the postures.

This is all that is necessary as a daily routine. The postures and breathing exercises can be done in about 15 minutes. You can take longer when you are more proficient at some of the postures, but it may then be better to do only three postures a day, covering the six in two days. To this 15 minutes you will add the time you decide to give for meditation, say 15 minutes to make a total of half an hour.

The remaining lessons give a few more postures but these are meant to be alternatives to the above basic six.

C. **Breathing**

Remember that in the *bellows breath* and the *throat cleansing breath* (lesson 2) you can take twice as long to exhale as to inhale.

(7) *Prana breathing*

According to the Indian tradition prana is the Life Principle at all levels of consciousness and is popularly translated as "the breath of life" (see also lesson 2). At the physical level it is the vital energy associated with the act of breathing, which sustains the link between the life of the body and life of the cosmos.

Pranayama is the control of the breath and, by this, the control of all life energies. It is therefore something more than the taking in of oxygen through the lungs, it is the absorption of the vital energy by the subtle counterpart of the physical body (sometimes called the etheric double) from the surrounding "psychic atmosphere". The following exercise, is for the conscious control of this prana intake.

Breathe slowly and normally while lying flat on the back. After three or four breaths feel that the air (with its vitality, prana) is coming in through the arms, legs, spine and head, and out the same way. In other words, as you breathe in, take in prana over the whole etheric body; when breathing out expel prana over the whole etheric body. This revitalizes the whole health aura and can revive a drooping etheric. The term etheric refers to the subtle vital counterpart of the dense physical body.

D. Meditation

For this lesson the exercise on prana breathing given above, can take the place of the meditation after the postures.

LESSON 8

This lesson deals with the chakras which were introduced in lesson 7 and takes prana breathing a stage
further. It also explains the different postures for meditation.

B. Postures

Having by now loosened up the body by the various
postures, you may now wish to adopt more advanced
postures for some of the breathing exercises and for
meditation. In lesson 2, under breathing, the Lotus
pose was described simply as "cross-legged", and the
Egyptian pose as on a chair with legs and feet together,
spine upright.

You may decide that, for you, the Egyptian pose is
more satisfactory. If this is so, the following postures
may be ignored. They are, however, recommended for
the advanced practice of Hatha Yoga, but it would be
unwise to force them, as an uncomfortable position will
undo any good the posture should give. It is far better
to use the Egyptian pose and concentrate on the breathing and meditation than to spoil the latter by an uncomfortable Lotus pose.

There are three principle "Lotus" poses, although it
is only the third (padmāsana) which is strictly the Lotus
posture.

(8) *Simple cross-legged posture* (sukhāsana)
The literal translation is "the pleasant seat".

Sit on a rug with the legs out in front. Bend the left

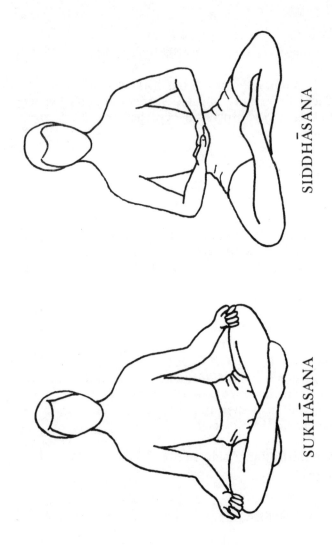

SIDDHĀSANA

SUKHĀSANA

42

leg at the knee and place the left foot under the right *thigh*, sole upwards and with the left knee as near the ground as possible. Do not worry if your knee cannot touch the ground.

Now bend the right leg at the knee and place the right foot under the left *leg*, sole tilted up. Note that for this simple posture the right foot is under the left leg, not the left thigh. The knees will probably be 4 to 6 inches from the ground.

Keep the body erect and extend the arms outwards to rest the back of the wrists on the knees.

Some people prefer to reverse the order, i.e. to have the right foot under the left thigh for the first movement.

The above description is rather detailed. If you find it easy to sit cross-legged on the ground, then ignore these instructions and just take the most comfortable position for yourself, so long as you keep the body erect.

The position of the hands is that for an "open meditation". For a "closed meditation" the hands may rest centrally one on the other palms up, or with the fingers interlaced.

(9) *Advanced cross-legged posture* (siddhāsana)
Literal translation—"the adept's seat".

Begin as for simple cross-legged. Bend the left knee and, with the help of the right hand, place the left heel under the centre of the pelvis (the perineum). The sole of the left foot will then be touching the inside of the right thigh.

Now bend the right knee, lift the right foot over the left leg and fit the toes snugly into the crevice between the calf and thigh of the left leg.

The position is similar to the simple one but more tightly held, and with the knees definitely resting on the ground. The right foot is higher, its upper surface resting inverted on the left calf.

Hands are now usually held together, palms up, right on left.

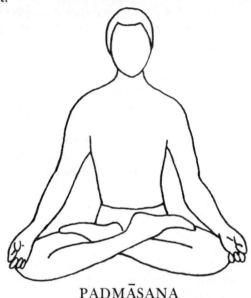

PADMĀSANA

(10) *Lotus Posture* (padmāsana)
Literally "the lotus seat".

This is the most difficult and not regarded as suitable for western people. You may, however, wish to know how it is done in case you are young enough to try it. Put briefly, the feet are pulled up so that their top surfaces, inverted, rest on the thighs.

44

Begin with the feet out in front. Bend the left knee and bring the heel under the centre of the pelvis as for the advanced posture. Then bring the right foot over the left thigh in an inverted position. Thus the sole of the left foot rests against the underside of the right thigh, while the top of the right foot rests on the top of the left thigh. This is the simple form of the lotus posture.

For the full lotus posture the left foot is pulled between the calf and thigh of the right leg so that the tops of both feet rest on the tops of the thighs. It is easier if the left foot is placed on the right thigh before positioning the right foot.

The hands are then rested on the knees. An official position is to have the hands, palms upwards and with the thumb and forefinger forming a circle, but many people prefer to have the palms downwards on the knees or thighs.

C. Breathing

(8) *Chakra breathing*

Just as prana may be taken in through the whole of the body and limbs as described in the last lesson (prana breathing), so it can also be taken in through any one of the occult centres (chakras). Chakra breathing is used by experienced yogis to awaken or to stimulate the nerve centres corresponding with the chakras. It is particularly a practice of Laya Yoga (see Introduction), but it is also used by Hatha yogis and therefore some details are required in this course.

It is assumed that, if you are interested, you will have studied the books on the chakras mentioned in the last lesson. As a general recommendation we do not advise the practice of chakra breathing except under careful supervision and then only by those who have a well-established control of their behaviour, mental, emotional and physical.

The method is to sit as for meditation using one of the postures described in this lesson, or in the Egyptian pose. Breathe normally but slowly, two or three times. Then switch attention to the site of the chakra and, while breathing in, try to visualize prana entering your system through that chakra. As you breathe out think of this prana vitalizing that particular chakra and spreading to the whole system with the special quality of the chakra chosen.

This should be done only once a day and never for more than 4 minutes.

The location of the seven principal chakras was given in the last lesson. We do not recommend the stimulation of any chakra below the heart and it is necessary to give the warning that any chakra breathing can bring about physical or nervous disturbances unless well controlled and supervised. You may, however, use a very limited form, say just one or two breaths, to bring the harmony of the higher worlds into the consciousness of the lower self using the following correspondences.

The *brow chakra*, at our present stage of evolution, corresponds to the higher Self or that part of our consciousness which may be called the "illumined mind". In Theosophy this is referred to as buddhi-manas: buddhi is the harmonizing principle, manas in this context is the higher mind. Buddhi is sometimes called the intuition, but wisdom is a better translation. Manas literally means the mind but it is always associated either with buddhi (the life of the Spirit) or with desire (Sanskrit, kāma). Thus buddhi-manas is the higher mind

46

illumined by the Self; kāma-manas is the lower mind which forms the personal and desire nature of man.

Meditation on the brow chakra therefore raises our consciousness to the level of the Spirit, man's higher Self and brings peace and harmony. Breathing prana through this chakra prepares the nervous system to receive that harmonizing influence.

The *throat chakra* corresponds to the bridge between higher Self and so-called lower self. It more particularly represents the path or bridge (Sanskrit antahkarana = instrument between) between the higher and lower mind and so it is the link between the divine Ego and the personal soul of man.

Thought on this chakra and breathing prana through it helps to channel the life of the higher Self into the physical body so that its activity may be controlled by selfless motives. Speech is centred at the throat and, since this chakra is the line of communication between higher and lower self (spirit and matter), we see the importance of control of speech, that it may express nothing to hurt or injure others, nor betray the speaker into irresponsible words and actions.

The *heart chakra* represents the highest level of the personal self. Just as the heart controls the life blood, so the corresponding chakra is the link for the lower mind to control desire and action. (See reference to kama-manas above.)

In books on meditation we find such expressions as "Feel peace in the heart", "The heart of the self-controlled man draws the hearts of all men into his heart", "The Self within my heart is one with all other selves". Breathing prana through this chakra is said to make man instinctively aware of the joys and sorrows of others.

There are three chakras below the heart: the solar plexus corresponding to the emotional nature, the spleen corresponding to the etheric or vital counterpart of the physical body and the root (at the base of the spine) representing the dense physical body itself. Since yoga is a process to realize one's identity with the Supreme, these lower centres should not be directly stimulated because this would give undue emphasis to the personal nature rather than to the higher spiritual Self. To control and direct the lower self it is quite sufficient to do this from the heart, corresponding to the highest principle of that lower self. Remember that the expression "from the heart" has both a literal meaning, i.e. from the heart chakra and a mystical meaning, i.e. from the love principle.

LESSON 9

B. Postures

(11) *Shoulder stand* (sarvāngāsana)

The Sanskrit word means the posture of all the limbs and it is therefore regarded as the basic posture. It stretches the whole body.

i. Lie flat on your back on a folded blanket or thick rug, legs together and arms at the sides, palms down. Slowly elevate the legs until they are vertical to the ground. Pause momentarily.

ii. Then press the hands and elbows on the floor and slowly raise the legs, hips, body and back. Finally, slide the hands up to press on the small of the back as a support from the elbows. (The palms are now upwards.) Your legs will swing beyond the vertical over the head at an angle of about 45°.

iii Finally give the body an extra lift with the hands to bring the trunk vertical and then bring the legs back to

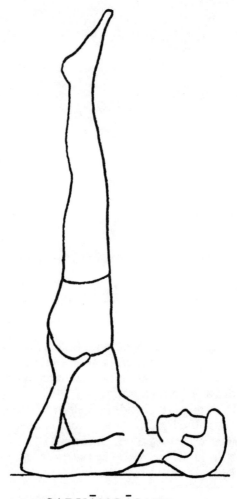

SARVĀNGĀSANA

the vertical. You are now in one straight line upside down from your shoulders.

The aim is to retain position iii for 2–3 minutes, and then to return *slowly* to the floor, keeping the full stretch throughout. You will already have achieved i in the plough posture, lesson 6, so proceed to ii in the first place, then to iii for just a few seconds. Then try to hold iii for half a minute and so on to a normal of 2 minutes or a maximum of 4 minutes.

At a later stage in your training you can combine the plough with the shoulder stand. Do the shoulder stand first to position iii. After holding that for the specified time, proceed to stages ii and iii of the plough posture (see lesson 6) and hold that for up to 30 seconds before returning to relax flat on the floor.

You now have eleven postures from which to choose nine for daily practice:

Before the breathing exercises, *relaxation* B 1
With the breathing exercises, *cross-legged* B 8, 9 or 10
After the breathing exercises, *back-stretching* B 2
twist B 3
shoulder stand B 11
plough B 4
bow B 5
cobra B 6
hand and foot B 7

If pressed for time you can omit B 2 and combine B 11 and B 4.

Further postures given in this and the next lesson are supplementary to the basic course, and can be used later by way of variety.

(12) *Abdominal uplift* (uddīyānā bandha)

The true yogic tradition puts the bandhas in a different category from the āsanas. They are "holds", "controls" or "locks". The word bandha literally means bondage. This particular bandha holds the whole abdominal area inward and upward as if by a natural corset. The Sanskrit word uddīyānā means "pulling up".

Stand with the knees slightly bent and hands on thighs palms down. Breathe in and out deeply, longer each time, finally exhaling as fully as possible. Then pull the abdomen in as far as possible, and upward. This is helped by raising the chest (lungs empty). Hold for 5 seconds only, then inhale and relax.

Repeat once only.

The Indian yogis hold the position for up to 1 minute or longer. It is said to prevent constipation. The exercise is not recommended if commenced over 50 years of age.

As a variant the pull-back and up can be made towards the right or the left.

Incidentally this bandha is one which can be done while in bed.

C. Breathing

(9) *Cooling breath* (sitakari)

This is an optional extra for special use. It is claimed to cure insomnia and can be used in hot weather to produce a cooling effect. Breathe in through the teeth with a hissing noise and out through the nose, ten times.

Open the lips but keep the teeth together. Hold the tongue so that the tip is just behind the lower teeth. Let air come in sharply as a cooling breath.

Then close the lips and breathe out through the nostrils.

After some practice the speed can be increased.

(10) There is another breathing exercise also called a *cooling breath* (sitali) but in this case the tongue protrudes out through the lips to suck the air in. The particular value of sitali is to clear the sinuses. Withdraw the tongue and close the lips to breathe out. Do this ten times.

Comment on throat cleansing breath (C 4, lesson 2)

This breath stimulates the throat chakra (see lesson 8). It also removes phlegm from the throat and helps such conditions as asthma and bronchitis.

D. Meditation

Daily meditation should now become a regular routine after the Hatha Yoga exercises. If you have meditated regularly before beginning this course, then you should have no problems and can continue with the method with which you are familiar. If the idea of a regular meditation is new to you, then you will require to follow the recommendations to be found in textbooks on the subject.

For the person experienced in meditation as well as for the beginner, the following should be noted:

Learn the value of silence.

Once every day examine your motives and reasons for your actions.

To banish fears, however minor, draw up a list of these, with the logical conclusions and then burn it.

If you make a shopping list, try leaving it at home.

Try not to jump to conclusions. When questioned, *think* and then reply.

You will note from the above suggestions that the idea is to use the value of meditation throughout the day and not just at the period of the official daily meditation. The suggestions in the meditation sections of lessons 1 and 4 were made with the same idea and should be read again.

For the beginner it has been explained in lesson 4 that this course will not deal with the practice of meditation in detail. It has purposely been limited to Hatha Yoga practices. Meditation is such an important subject that it requires a special course on its own. It is strongly recommended that you consider this and put yourself in a position to be able to include a set meditation with other yoga exercises. For recommended books on the subject see lesson 4.

If, after experience, you find you are not the "meditating type", you should still conclude the other yoga exercises with a period of quietness. The whole object of all yoga practices is to raise the consciousness above the level of ordinary acting, feeling and thinking. The Raja yogi seeks to bring all thinking processes to a standstill so that the light from above may shine unimpeded to illumine all activity below. This leads to a transcendence of the limits of ordinary consciousness as it merges into superconsciousness. Such is the ideal.

If you cannot undertake the necessary special training to acquire such technique, you can at least move in that direction by making the process a little less mental. Just sit still without making the mind do anything. Teach the body to become unaware of all the little itches and irritations which draw attention to themselves. Do this for 5 minutes, and repeat it next day, and the next and so on until you really can control the body and make it rest comfortably. Then proceed to calm the feelings, the emotions; stop worrying, stop disliking things or people. Feel love and acceptance of your environment.

Then, when you can sit quietly and peacefully, is the time to start to train the mind to think calmly and one-pointedly. It may be at this stage that you feel you are not the meditating type. What such a feeling really means, is that you may not be the mental meditating type.

In that case take a subject such as beauty, harmony, truth or any other quality which appeals to you. Use it as something to brood on rather than to think about. Such an approach can lead to a state of oneness with the inspiration, not in an intellectual way, but as a calm restrained self-realization which can become a mighty force to be used in the service of the Highest.

The important thing about meditation, whatever one's best method of approach, is to remember that persistent repetition of pure emotions and good thoughts must rebuild the individual's mental and emotional principles along the lines of the chosen ideal.

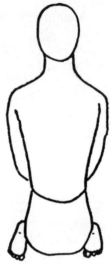

VAJRĀSANA

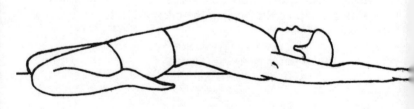

SUPTA-VAJRĀSANA

LESSON 10

This is the last lesson and should therefore be a time for revision. Read through all the lessons again to get them into proper perspective and to consider how much you have achieved. The only additional items in this lesson are four more postures. This does not mean that you have to increase the time given daily for these exercises. The new ones should be used as alternatives and to introduce variety.

You should decide how much of the whole Course you wish to adopt and then plan your future routine in such a way that you *use the system* without being used by it. At the end of this lesson a suggested programme is given to serve as a guide.

B. Postures

(13) *Pelvic posture* (supta-vajrāsana)

Kneel, with the knees together, the feet about 12 inches apart, soles upward, and sit between the feet. Begin with the spine upright (vajrāsana) and then bend backwards until the spine rests on the floor with the arms stretched back.

This stretches the thigh muscles and the abdomen and so may be used occasionally instead of the bow posture. (B 5, lesson 6.)

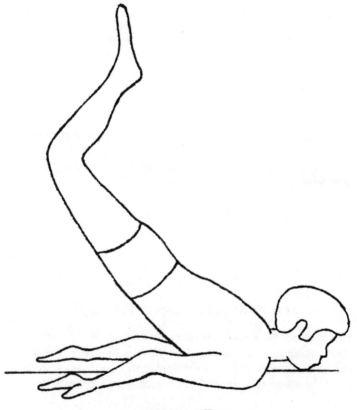

SHALABHĀSANA

(14) *Locust posture* (shalabhāsana)

This is an exceptional posture in that it requires a sudden movement. Lie face down with arms at the side, hands palms down, elbows slightly bent (fingers pointing towards the feet). Then suddenly raise the legs and thighs (and body if possible) off the ground. Only the chin, shoulders and chest should touch the ground. Hold the position for only 1 second.

This is like the cobra posture but raising the feet instead of the head. It can therefore be used, occasionally only, instead of the cobra. (B 6, lesson 7.)

In the introduction to this course the position of Hatha Yoga relative to other forms of yoga was briefly outlined. It was suggested that Jnana, Bhakti, Karma and Raja Yogas were superior to the others, and that Hatha Yoga should be taken as supplementary. If you did not begin this Course after some work on one of the other yogas, it is hoped that you will have been inspired to wish to take up one of the above four, preferably Raja. Suggestions have been given for the use of meditation in your daily practice and books on the subject were recommended in lesson 4. If you now wish to cover a still wider range, the following books are recommended:

Yoga, Ernest Wood.

The Science of Yoga, I. K. Taimni.

Raja Yoga, A Simplified and Practical Course, Wallace Slater.

Raja-Yoga, Jnana-Yoga, Bhakti-Yoga and *Karma-Yoga* (4 books), Vivekananda.

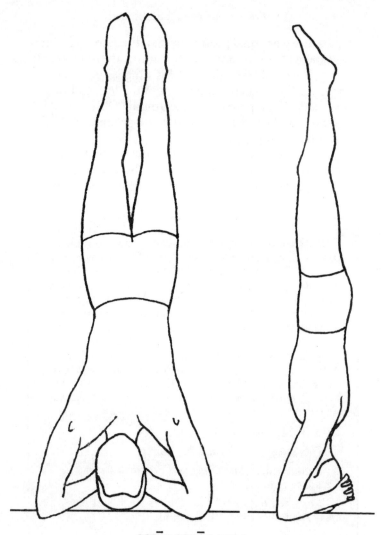

SHĪRSHĀSANA

60

(15) *Head stand* (shīrshāsana)

This posture requires personal instruction and great care. The following is a general description of how it is carried out. It is called the head stand but the inverted body is actually supported on the forearms as well as the head.

Kneel down, lean forward and put the head and forearms on the ground. Then gradually raise the body and legs (knees bent) into the vertical upside-down position. This may require the assistance of another person in the first place, and later it should be done against a wall. Then straighten the legs.

You can remain in this position for up to 5 minutes, but proceed carefully to avoid giddiness. In fact it may be necessary not to proceed beyond the first stage of putting the head and forearms on the ground. See how you feel like this—do not go further until you can be sure you have no giddy sensation.

As this is an upside-down posture it can be used instead of the shoulder stand. (B 11, lesson 9.)

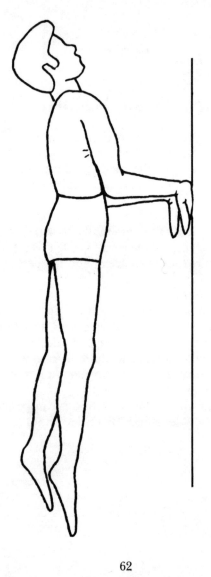

MAYŪRĀSANA

(16) *Peacock posture* (mayūrāsana)

Kneel with the knees about 12 inches apart. Place the hands, palms down on the floor about 18 inches in front of the knees with the wrists to the front. Bend forward until the abdomen is resting on the elbows. Then raise the body and legs to a horizontal position with the legs outstretched as a letter V. The horizontal body is now resting on the hands with the forearms vertical. Hold the position for a few seconds only.

This posture is very good for the digestive organs and can cure piles. It is not suited to women.

D. Meditation

You can use a meditation period as an exercise to solve a problem.

i. First collect the facts about the problem, e.g. suppose you have a difficulty which you have to meet today, tomorrow or next week.

ii. Then ask yourself what is the worst possible result that can happen, and decide to accept even this if necessary.

iii. Then dismiss the problem from your mind but with the hope and the expectation of a good result.

iv. Then relax for the intuition to work.

Many dilemmas can be solved in this way, Stage i is most important. If done thoroughly it will avoid the emotional personal result which so many people claim as divine inspiration.

Typical daily programme

The following will be found to "flow easily" and takes about half an hour each morning.

(1) Relaxation posture   (B 1, lesson 1)

(2) Breathing exercises

Basic breath	(C 1, lesson 1)
Head cleansing breath	(C 2, lesson 2)
Bellows breath	(C 3, lesson 2)
Throat cleansing breath	(C 4, lesson 2)
Empty breath	(C 5, lesson 3)
Full breath	(C 6, lesson 3)

(3) Postures

Back-stretching	(B 2, lesson 4)
Twist	(B 3, lesson 5)
Plough	(B 4, lesson 6)
Shoulder stand	(B 11, lesson 9)
Bow	(B 5, lesson 6)
Cobra	(B 6, lesson 7)
Hand and foot	(B 7, lesson 7)

(4) Meditation

(1) and (2) will take say	9 minutes
(3) ,, ,, ,,	6 minutes
(4) should take	15 minutes
Total	30 minutes

"The laws of evolution of consciousness in the universe are exactly the same as the laws of Yoga, and the principles whereby consciousness unfolds itself in the great evolution of humanity are the same principles as we take in Yoga and deliberately apply to the more rapid unfolding of our own consciousness."

ANNIE BESANT

"With the sword of my will, I carve for myself a throne in the realm of the Spirit, which I shall ascend."

N. SRI RAM